STAYING *in* RHYTHM *with the* LION *of the* TRIBE *of* JUDAH!

A BOOK WRITTEN BY *Holy Spirit*
THROUGH *A. Vessels*

STAYING *in* RHYTHM
with the LION *of the* TRIBE *of* JUDAH!

A BOOK WRITTEN BY *Holy Spirit*
THROUGH *A. Vessels*

XULON PRESS

Xulon Press
2301 Lucien Way #415
Maitland, FL 32751
407.339.4217
www.xulonpress.com

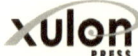

Unless otherwise indicated, Scripture quotations taken from the King James Version (KJV) – *public domain.*

Printed in the United States of America.

ISBN-13: 978-1-54565-121-6

Staying in Rhythm
with the Lion of the Tribe of Judah

THANKSGIVING

Lord, I thank you for what you have entrusted me to do. I am humbled and privileged to be available to you to train, encourage, and build your body. Who would have thought that you would take something like physical fitness, more specifically bodybuilding, and use it for your kingdom's sake? I know that you knew all along; however, this new thing that you are causing to spring up in me wows me. Once again, thank you Abba Father.

TABLE OF CONTENTS

Introduction

Life is the quality that distinguishes a vital, functional plant or animal from a dead body—a state of living, characterized by the capacity for metabolism, growth, reaction to stimuli, and reproduction. This is what a dictionary defined life to be. Another defines it only as: the existence of an individual human being or animal.

I personally have a larger revelation on the definition of what that word *life* means. That word is "The Word," He is Life. "The Word became flesh, and dwelt among us and we beheld His glory, the glory as the only begotten of the Father." John 1:14. "I am the way, the truth, and the life. No man comes to the Father, but by me." John 14:6 "He that hath the Son hath life; and he that hath not the Son hath not life." 1 John 5:12

That is plain enough for me. I receive that as truth; however, there was a time that I had to push the boundaries. I couldn't hear truth because I just did not have ears to hear it, nor did I have a will or desire to obey it. I still push boundaries, but to the increase of life. Light that is also life, to dispel darkness; this is now my desire. I am, indeed, in the process of being changed, the Lord is faithful, and He will complete the work that He has begun in me.

In Jeremiah 1:4-5, we see God the Father enlightening Jeremiah as to his calling. In verse 5, "Before I formed thee in the belly, I knew thee; and, before thou camest forth out of the womb, I sanctified thee, and ordained thee a prophet unto the nations."

So, we see here that God the Father had a plan, as well as a design, before Jeremiah ever came to be. If the Father has a plan for us from the womb and all, then, what happens to us? Why are there so many of us wondering, "What am I here for? What is the meaning of this whole thing called life?" The answer is simple. We were born into this earth.

Now I'm not coming from a "Woe is me for being born" point of view. I'm stating a mere fact here. We see it in Psalms 51:5, "Behold, I was shapen in iniquity; and in sin did my mother conceive me." Psalms 58:3, "The wicked are estranged from the womb: they go astray as soon as they be born, speaking lies." Sounds a bit intense—especially for a baby; however, this is the fact. Truth is solid, facts are subject to change.

We were formed in our mother's womb by God and came into this world and began to acquire mountains of information. We are bombarded with information on how to be, what love is, how to express it, what a woman does—or does not do, what a man is or is not, what, how, who, and blah, blah. Taking in all of that information without proper guidance, some of us have lost our perception on a few things, that is if we ever had a clear perception to begin with.

It has always grieved me, in my spirit, when I hear a person ask, what happened to someone who is down, or merely existing. We get an answer: LIFE happened. Life does not happen to you; it is a gift.

I took a course once where the instructor started one of her lectures with, "Life is just one big problem after another. You solve one and then you are on to the next." *Really?* That's it? I want to shed some light on that subject: Jesus said in John 10:10, "The thief comes not, but for to steal, and to kill, and to destroy: I am come that they might have life, and that they may have it more abundantly." It is the cares and worries of this world that want to weigh us down, as burdens, to choke out life. This is what we have seen happening to people.

I recently went to a worship conference and heard a young lady teach a message on being what God has created us to be. This sounds simple, but the delivery of it was quite profound. She spoke on how sometimes people can become so gripped with fear that they just can't move forward into what God the Father has formed and led them to be. This can happen if we replace God's plan for us with a negative frame of mind, such as: doubt, feelings of unworthiness, shame, or self-pity.

She basically called God's plan for our lives *Plan A.* Anything other than this choice is less than His plan. We can call the lesser choices: *Plan B, C,* or *D*, or however long we choose to make the list of alternate options.

The truth is that, if we are not doing what we were created to do, we won't be content. The fearful and wonderful configuration of God's will always yields this yearning to become what He has formed us to be, and to walk in it. It's like an ache that cannot be satisfied by any natural means.

Chapter 1

THE ASSIGNMENT

D id you know that if your heart is not perfectly aligned with the heart of God the Father, you can't hear Him? That's really a lie, please don't stop reading. I will tell you that I truly had a reverential fear to even write that lie; however, we are taking a view behind the enemy's camp and I believe that it will help some of us. There are so many people who have believed lies like this. We've believed imaginations like, *we have to get our sins in order before we can come to God* or that, *we are too wretched for God the Father to want us.* We can't get sins in order without God. We need the blood of Jesus, we need His help, His direction. Really, no man comes unto Jesus except when the Father places that desire in his heart by Holy Spirit. It is His love, mercy, and goodness that will induce conviction in us, to a repentant heart.

There is not a dungeon, dark corner, or distance where one can exist that the Father can't reach. We just have to come to grips with the truth that it is His way, and not ours, and that God the Father does not see things as man does. It is as the palmist David spoke of our Father: "Whither shall I go from thy Spirit, or whither shall I flee from thy presence? If I ascend up into the heaven, thou art there; If I make my bed in hell, behold, Thou art there. If I take the wings of the morning, and dwell in the uttermost parts of the sea, even there shall Thy hand lead me, and Thy right hand shall hold me." Psalms 139 7-10. I person-ally know that I know this is true.

Back in the nineties, I lived in Cancun, México. I had been a personal trainer for many years and had danced since the age of eight. While I lived in Mexico, I personally trained people, taught hip hop to girls from age six to eight, and English as a second language to adults. There was a school called Harmon Hall where I taught English. I taught dance at a studio called Cima, and I personally trained people at Gold's gym.

The sun shone brightly, and it was hot most of the year in Cancun; so, people were in their summer get-in-shape mode all year round. This really worked well for me. I stayed busy, with my day beginning in the early morning until noon, siesta, and then back at four until evening. Business was good with clients coming in every hour on the hour. The hand of God was on me and, indeed, held me. I will tell you now that, at that time, I did not seek that my heart would be in line with the Father's at all. For that reason, my walk with Him went astray.

I had a deeper relationship with Him before this time; how-ever, there were some cares that I began to look at and med-itate on. My vision and my perception on things had become skewed. In that time of my life, my idea of communing with Abba Father was sitting down and reading a page from "My utmost for His Highest," a daily devotional by Oswald Chambers. I said, "reading a page." I did not say anything about listening to Abba Father. Even in my diminished view of our relation-ship and time of intimacy, He never stopped reaching for me, and His right hand held me. Now, if a page from a devotional is your time of intimacy with the Father, I do not say this by any means as a slight to you, or your relationship with Him. It is just that I have come to know He has so much more that He wants to share with us.

As I said, clients came in on the hour, and one day, this client arrived and wanted to just talk with me. Although she was scheduled to train, we just talked, and as the conversation went on, things got pretty deep. She began to share about some areas in which she definitely needed healing. Some were concerning tragic family loss and relationships. As I look back now, I see there were some areas where her perception on some things had become skewed and she held onto these perceptions very tightly. Now I have a better understanding of what I was seeing, but then it was hard to comprehend. Similar things happened with a few other clients in a short time of instruction from Holy Spirit. Although I had my own selfish, worldly agenda and was following it with great tenacity, I recognized the unction of the Spirit of God and began to pay attention to what He was showing me. I knew in my spirit that the things I saw at that time went beyond just the natural. They were natural circumstances; but the Holy Ghost had a supernatural instruction for me.

I remember one day in the gym after one of those conversations with a client, I placed my hands on my hips and asked the Lord out loud, "What is going on?" The Lord responded right then and there, "There is a need!" *Wow.* I felt this answer with my whole being. I remember telling the Lord that He was going to have to help me because I didn't know what to do. I knew enough about counseling to know that you don't just open up Pandora's Box without being prepared to deal with what comes out. The issues that these people were sharing were deep and intense. I did not feel prepared at all, but even so, I accepted the assignment by asking the Father for His help.

If you have received Jesus as your Savior, there is always a process of some sort in Him. We are constantly being transformed from glory to glory into the image of Christ.

Right now, you may be in a difficult part of a process...or even what seems to be a barren wilderness. When Holy Spirit comes to intervene, intercept, or even arrest a development that is not the Father's heart for you, that is not His *plan A* for you, harden not your heart. There have been so many of us walking in *plan F*, to maybe *plan M* and so on, because when the Holy Spirit came to deliver, redirect, and instruct us there was a hardening of heart. I've been there, and I have done that! People sometimes begin to look at themselves when God shines light on the very thing that He wants to deliver them from. Sometimes pride rises up because we may think that we should be better than that, or we feel exposed, or even spiritually lacking. The truth is, "Blessed are the poor in spirit, for theirs is the kingdom of heaven." Matthew 5:3. If we will walk in the truth that we are in need of our Savior 24/7/365, we will welcome His correction and instruction with open arms. We will recognize the Kingdom of God coming to us at that moment and receive it.

> We must remember: "Our Father who art in heaven, hallowed be Thy name. Thy kingdom come. Thy will be done in earth, as it is in heaven. give us this day our daily bread. and forgive us our debts, as we forgive our debtors. and lead us not into temptation, but DELIVER US FROM EVIL: for Thine is the kingdom, and all the power, and the glory for ever. Amen." Matthew 6:9-13

In this manner, we have been instructed to pray. Deliverance is the Kingdom of God coming to us. It is His life and truth coming to us and our being made free. The Holy Ghost brings the light and life of Jesus Christ, however He deems necessary so that we walk not in darkness. We must not let our hearts become stony when the Holy Spirit shines LIGHT on the matter.

Chapter 2

SHE CAN BE TAUGHT!

J ust this morning before starting this chapter, I felt a leading from Holy Spirit to stay still. It was not intense just, a gentle "be still." To be honest with you, I really did not know what that looked like, or what to do except be still, or to do nothing. I even said to myself that if anyone wanted me to do anything this day, I would tell them that this is what I felt led to do. Shortly after, a friend left me a voice mail that she was going to go out of town at five in the evening and she was inviting me to go. I started to ponder the idea; thinking that by that time, I would have been still most of the day. Maybe it would be okay for me to go by then. I didn't ask Holy Spirit; I just tried to start leaning. In Proverbs 3:5-6, our instructions are: "Trust in the Lord with all thine heart and lean not unto thine own understanding. In all thy ways acknowledge Him, and He shall direct thy path."

One time when I read that scripture, Holy Spirit gave me an actual visual understanding on it. I saw a stick person leaning backwards on one heel of one foot. The other leg of this character was forward in the air; it was about to fall. The Spirit of God knows that if I see, I will remember. It's just how I am wired.

He was showing me that, if a person leans to his own understanding, he would be setting himself up for a fall. I truly believe this, especially when God the Father has given them a directive.

A person, at that point, may have come into agreement with pride saying that they know better than God. Proverbs 16:18 shows us that: "Pride goeth before destruction and an haughty spirit before a fall."

I remember an occasion where I received a word of warning from the Lord out of the mouth of three of His witnesses; these were people that I know hear from Him. They all said the same thing in a different way and at different times. I, on the other hand, had *leaned on my own understanding* of some things that the Lord had shown me about the same matter. Although the things that I saw were from the Lord, I did not ask Him what I was seeing or what it meant. This is where the problem was. I did not acknowledge Him in it. I leaned and fell, and oh, how hard was the fall.

When God made male and female, He told them to subdue the earth and have dominion over it. The desire for us to rule, govern, and exercise authority is from God. This is how He created us and what He told us to do from the beginning. Our being in Him and our seeking that our hearts be in line with the Father's heart are crucial for His Kingdom to come and His will to be done through us in the earth. We have to remember that perception thing. If we don't recognize and understand the position that God has given us on His earth, we won't appreciate, respect, or honor it. We could say that about every gift that has come down from the Father. We could insert: family, friends, spouses, spiritual gifts, talents, or money...the list goes on. How we perceive ourselves, others, and things has everything to do with how we will respond. How we perceive the Holy Spirit has everything to do with our response to Him.

I remember one morning last year when the Holy Spirit said, "You have to come to the place where you believe me, no matter what." He then took me on a few lessons up close and personal. I would be driving and suddenly He would tell me to turn in somewhere and do something. On two occasions, it looked like I had missed Him altogether. I will share one; the Holy Spirit told me to make a hoodie with a slogan on it. He had been telling me to do this for a minute; however, I dragged my feet. One day He said, "Go make that shirt." Immediately I turned that truck onto the street of the establishment where the hoodie was to be made. When I got inside the business, I asked the lady behind the counter if they had any lightweight hoodies. Before I could really get the question out of my mouth, she gave me a sharp, "No." I asked about her venders, and she quickly said they didn't have any. Now this is a company that prints on shirts, and it was about to be the springtime of the year; I was not asking for the unlikely. I stood there remembering what Holy Spirit told me to do and then recapped what the woman had just told me. It looked like I had missed Him altogether.

When the design of this shirt came to me it was a lightweight hoodie, I really wanted to follow His instruction. Suddenly the owner of the business came out from the back and said, "I thought that I saw some lightweight hoodies right over here this weekend." The woman who'd told me *no* came out from behind the counter and followed the owner saying, "No I sold them." At this point, I had disconnected from the nay sayer and focused on someone who was trying to help me. The owner found not one, not two, but three of the style that I was looking for right there in the store. The whole time the other attendant was standing there saying that there were not any there. Wow! If I had not believed the Holy Spirit, I would have walked out of that business the first time she'd said "No." If not walked out, then maybe compromised His instruction by going with a design different than what He showed me in the beginning. He knows what He is doing. It's a simple truth that can be applied to so many areas of our lives when the Holy Ghost is on the scene. He is the Spirit of truth, and He will teach us all things, He will also lead us into all truth.

The Holy Spirit continued with these instructional exercises, and some were costly when I leaned on my own understanding. I had a Doberman and wolf-mix breed of dog. She was a beautiful blue color with the most stunning eyes. She was about six months old. My family homestead is in between two hunting clubs. Every year from November to January, there were numerous hunters in those woods. Every year around that time I would kennel my dogs. About two Januarys ago, it was time to let them run free. The hunters were out of the woods. Esther, my beautiful blue pup had literally never run with the big dogs. When I let them out, she ran back and forth to me and to her dad, the wolf. The Holy Ghost said, "Don't let her go!" She kept running back to me then her dad. She looked so eager to go with him. I should have kept her with me, but I didn't. When the big dogs came back from their run, Esther was missing from the pack. Day in and day out I looked for her. I hoped that possibly she might navigate her way home or somewhere near. She didn't. There were other similar lessons; I finally got it.

I always saw the Holy Spirit as my comforter. I knew that He is the Spirit of truth but did not so much depend on Him to lead me. In John 16:7, Jesus tells us: "Nevertheless I tell you the truth; it is expedient for you that I go away: for if I go not away, the Comforter will not come unto you; but if I depart, I will send Him unto you." Thank you, Jesus! In John 16:12, Jesus speaks of the Holy Spirit: "Howbeit when He, the Spirit of truth, is come, He will guide you into all truth: for He shall not speak of Himself; but whatsoever He shall hear, that shall He speak: and He will show you things to come." Wow, what a glorious gift from such a splendid Friend.

You see, we can't walk this walk in the Spirit of God unless we are filled with the Spirit of God. Jesus told His disciples that He would send them the Comforter. He also told them that the world did not know the Spirit of truth, but they knew Him because He dwelt with them. Jesus goes on to tell His disciples that the Comforter, "Shall be in them." John14:17. Now in 1 Corinthians 2:14, Paul explains to us: "That a natural man receiveth not the things of the Spirit of God: for they are foolishness unto him: neither can he know them, because they are spiritually discerned." The Holy Spirit reveals unto us the things of God the Father. Holy Spirit searches and reveals the depth of Abba Father to us. Now how wonderful is that?

Chapter 3

JUST WHO ARE THESE SONS OF GOD?

I remember an experience that I had in the congregation of a church in Corrigan, Texas. My son and I attended this congregation on Wednesday nights, which was the night when they had youth ministry. It was an awesome time in the presence of the Lord for the youth, and my son loved it. They would worship and seek the Lord in their own radical ways, and the Holy Spirit would show up and bring whatever the Father wanted them to have at that time. It was so important to me for my son to know how to reach the Father for himself. We eventually became members of that congregation.

Corrigan First Assembly had experienced revival for some months before we got there, and this continued for some years after. It was a life-changing experience for me. During one of the meetings of this revival, someone mentioned *the sons of God* while ministering. I honestly don't remember who it was, but I do remember what the Holy Spirit did when I heard it. One scripture this minister spoke from was Romans 8:14, "For as many are led by the Spirit of God, they are the sons of God." He spoke of the earnest expectation of the creature waiting for the manifestation of the sons of God. Something happened in my spirit when I heard this word that night. The Lord did something in me because every time I quoted that scripture or heard it there was a resonating like an awakening alarm in my spirit. For as many as are led by the spirit of God, they are the sons of God. It got to the point that I would say it often because it would just well up and overflow out of me.

The youth group that my son was a part of went to Branded by Fire in Florida, so I had time to myself without too full of an agenda. I decided to fast and seek the Lord. I had been doing so, and, while praying in the Holy Ghost, the Lord began to show me a vision. I saw a person walking on the sand in a desert, where hills and sand dunes were around. At first, I couldn't tell who it was. The person had on what looked like a raw silk cloth covering her from foot to head. The only thing showing was the face, some of the head, and a little shoulder. It seemed as though this fabric was so close fitting, that it was like a restraint. As I continued to see, it looked like this cloth was similar to a cocoon and that this person was definitely coming out of it. As she was walking on this sandy way, I could see that she was in what seemed to be a sandstorm. She just continued to walk and this cocoon came off slowly because this sandstorm was blowing, like a grand exfoliation. By the Spirit of God, I sensed that the person was me. Once I began to look at the vision to write it out, a word in tongues came forth by Holy Spirit. Then the Lord gave me the interpretation: He said, "For I have set a course in motion within you, and you will see, and you will hear what I say. I have set a course. I have spoken and you have not always heard... you have not always hearkened," saith the Lord. "But from this day forward, you will see, and hear what exceeds from my mouth. I see your heart, and I have the reins."

Later in that same weekend, I was worshiping the Lord, praying, and seeking Him. He said quite loudly, "You speak of sonship! Do you know what that means? Do you know what that means?" It felt like a rebuke. I didn't say anything. My Abba is a loving Father, I know beyond a shadow of any doubt that He loves me. The Word shows us in Hebrews 12:5, "despise not thou the chastening of the Lord, nor faint when we are rebuked of Him." The Father knows our hearts. In this particular instance, He wanted me to grasp and know that there is so much more to walking in the authority that His Son came to give me. One of the things that the sacrifice of Christ established, is that we be heirs to the Kingdom of God and joint heirs with Christ Jesus. It is not a small thing. Abba Father did not want me to handle it lightly.

Although that was a definite rebuke, I have since felt the leading and aligning of my heart by Holy Spirit with the will and heart of Abba Father. The Father has ways that are so beyond our imagination. He is so grand and vast that we really can not fathom His thoughts without His Spirit; even then we see only in part. This is why, when the Holy Spirit tells us something, we need to pay attention. The Lord does not want us to just take a guess in the dark that He means this or that. He wants us to ask, to acknowledge Him, even about the things that He shows us. He will direct us. I have been taught and the teaching continues.

There is a thing here and it is that, no matter our age, we have to remain teachable. The Holy Ghost will teach us things that we know not when we remain teachable. We see in Exodus 3:2-5, that Moses is there on the back side of the desert, doing his thing when the Lord shows him a wondrous sight in the burning bush. In verse 4, the Bible shows us that when the Lord saw that Moses turned aside to see what He had put there to get his attention, was when the Lord began to give Moses some instructions that He had for his life.

Following instructions, doing things in a new or different way, submitting to authority all requires that we be *teachable*. We see in John 5:18-19, that the Jews of that day wanted to kill Jesus because He healed on the Sabbath. Basically, nothing about Jesus supported their mindset, their order, their anything. In their minds, Jesus was just not working for them or with them. Nevertheless, He said to them in verse 19, "The Son can do nothing of Himself, but what He seeth the Father do: for what things so ever He doeth, these also doth the Son likewise." Whoop! There it is! God's only begotten Son, Jesus, the Desire of the Nations did what He saw the Father do. He has made a provision that we can do the same by the Holy Spirit. How can we expect to LIVE this life without Jesus? How can we expect to do exploits without knowing Him and being led by Holy Spirit? In Daniel, we see that "many will do wickedly against the covenant of God: but the ones that know their God shall be strong, and do exploits." We have already established that this is by the Spirit of God who reveals to us the things of God.

Sometimes humans can have difficulty with change. A person may want what God has for them but have difficulty with letting go of their personal perception of it. Healing is change; deliverance is change; increase is change; learning to be led of the Spirit of the Almighty God is change. We are changed from glory to glory by the Spirit of the Lord. Where am I going with this? Jesus came and walked this walk before us. He has already made the way. It is by Holy Spirit that we shall do exploits in this earth or in whatever realm that He so desires. We must ask Him to teach us and then submit ourselves to life, which is Jesus, and live.

We have already established that we, as humans, want to rule and reign. That's okay as long as we are in Him and being led by His Spirit to do so. Jesus Himself was led into the wilderness by the Holy Ghost to be tempted of the devil. In Hebrews 4:14-16, verse 15 shows us: "We have not an high priest which cannot be touched with the feelings of our infirmities; but was in all points tempted like as we are, yet without sin." Verse 16 encourages us: "Let us therefore come boldly before the throne of grace, that we may obtain mercy, and find grace to help in a time of need." Jesus has come and done this thing for us. He has met humanity where we were as a whole and will meet you personally, exactly how you are individually.

When we do take a step to obey or believe whatever the Father says, then we watch His salvation begin to unfold in our being and the things that concern us. When the Holy Spirit tells us to do something, and we drag our feet, we are not obeying. Delayed obedience is still disobedience. When the Holy Spirit tells us to do something in a particular way, and we do it the way that feels most comfortable to us, once again we have dissed Him. When He tells us to do something, and it is not clear to us, we need to ask Him exactly how He wants it done. We need to ask Him. We don't want to jump in front of the Holy Spirit saying, "I know what to do, follow me!" The Holy Ghost is a leader, not a follower. I know from experience.

In Ephesians, He has called us to a circumspect walk. Let's look at other meanings of the word *circumspect*. God has called us to a watchful walk, attentive walk, and an alert walk, why? It matters where and how we place our feet. The Word tells us to be wise and understand what the will of the Lord is. We can only do this by His Spirit. "For as many as are led by the Spirit of God, they are the sons of God." "The Spirit itself beareth witness with our spirit, that we are the children of God." Romans 8:14, 16

Chapter 4

A PENNY FOR YOUR THOUGHTS

R emember in the beginning of these testimonies, I shared
that I had accepted the assignment of the Father, when I
told Him that He would have to help me because I didn't know
what to do with the things that I was seeing? Well, two years
after I asked Him for this help, I returned to the United States
from Mexico, and the Lord opened a door for me to go to school.
I attended a program for ground-level psych nursing in San
Bernardino, California.

It was a very intense program; I emphasize intense. It was
like these instructors put us in a blender and turned us all the
way up to puree, then watched to see what would happen with
us. There were two times, well into the program, in particular
that I wanted to quit or, should I say, I wanted them to back off.
I had meetings with instructors to negotiate the terms of the
program or, they met with me, to get me in line with it. It was
stressful, to say the least. In one such meeting with one of the
five instructors, she suggested that I withdraw from the program and come back the next year. What! There was no way
"in anything" that I would have come back to that. I told the
instructor that if I left then, I would not come back. The thought
of quitting after investing so much time, sweat, and tears was

more painful than the discomfort and stress of the program itself; hence, I resolved to continue.

Some of the stresses were things like, the program director speaking in broken English, because English was not her first language. If you called her office, you would hear her voice mail answer, "I am not on my desk right now, but if you leave me a message, I will get back to you as soon as possible." That's all good. I did understand that she meant that she was not at her desk; but this is how she wrote her tests! You would go in to take a test and not only have to figure out what she was asking, but you would also have to give the right answer. By all means, don't be late to class because then she would be on your heels, barking, before you took a 300-question test on *who knew what she was asking*.

There was another instructor who was not my favorite at all. This woman would say anything to you. I remember she had the class in a group therapy type of seating. We were in a circle. She slapped her desk with her hand and blurted out, "Ha! Imagine granny with her legs in the air!" I thought, "Oh my gosh, this can't be necessary. I don't want to imagine that!" She then just looked at us with no expression, observing our responses. The same woman said something to us that I remember to this day. She said, "When you lay down at night, put your thoughts in order." "In order, hmm, how do I do that?" I thought.

One instructor, near the end of the program— and yes, I did endure to the end by the grace and mercy of God alone—was reviewing various psychological disorders and emotional conditions. She brought out that, somewhere along the line, these disorders all began with fear.

These instructors were trying to prepare us to work with mentally-challenged patients or the criminally insane. They were trying to condition our minds and desensitize us to unhealthy or inappropriate social thinking. One reason for this was because some of the people that we would work with were not functioning in a healthy or appropriate social thought process. They also wanted to see if we could persevere or find out if we'd break during a moment of intensity or crisis.

You see...intensity, heat, pressure, and stress always let us know what we are made of. It just tends to come to the top. They pushed every button they could, to try to cause us to fear failing the program or fear in whatever way they could. Fears don't have to be of something actual; they can just be a matter of perception.

Saying this makes me think of when Goliath said to the armies of Israel, "I defy the armies of Israel this day give me a man that we may fight together." When Saul and all Israel heard those words of the Philistine, they were dismayed and greatly afraid. I understand that these men were afraid of an actual giant; however, here was David saying, "The Lord delivered me out of the paw of a lion and out of the paw of a bear; He will deliver me out of the hand of this Philistine." 1 Samuel 17:10, 37. David just perceived Goliath as another way for God to show Himself strong on his behalf. I flipped the script on the circumstance; however, David's perception on the situation made all the difference in the world. David did not focus on Goliath. His trust was in the Lord. In our eyes, these instructors were not our friends at all. Sometimes it seemed as though they were trying to make us fail. Every time we turned around, there was an issue. If they pushed a button and saw that it really got to us, it seemed as though they laid into that subject. They wanted to make us or break us. If we were going to break, I guess they felt in the program would be a better place than on a ward with the criminally insane or psychologically imbalanced. Sad to say, after this program, one of my classmates hung herself. Fear caused many to act out of character and the intensities of the situations were sometimes overwhelming. When I sat down to those tests, having no clue what this woman was saying because of obscure wording and knowing that I was guessing many times on a major test, I would cry myself into a meltdown. This was all a part of the program.

Believe it or not, the one instructor that was not my favorite, was actually one of the sweetest, most sensitive people I have ever met. She stood and made a speech at our student brunch. She wept and said that it always brought her joy to see students grow. I was able to talk to her after the brunch. I asked her, "What you guys are saying with all of this is that the clients are not going to change immediately...we have to." A big loving smile came across her face. She closed her eyes, nodded her head, and whispered, "Yes." At the end of the program, even the instructor who'd written those impossible-to-understand tests, the one who'd always been on my case, said to me, "I believe we deserve a hug."

There is another instructor who tries us, in order to bring about patience, to attain excellence in Him. Jesus desires to help us to endure and to overcome. In the book of James, in chapter 1, verse 3, we see, "Knowing this, that the trying of your faith worketh patience." What about James 1:12, where it is written, "Blessed is the man that endureth temptation: for when he is tried, he shall receive a crown of life, which the Lord hath promised to those that love Him." Look at 1 Peter 1:7, we see that: "The trial of your faith, being much more precious than of gold that perishes though it be tried with fire, might be found unto praise and honor and glory at the appearing of Jesus Christ." These tests are spiritual conditionings—exercises!

In the psych program, the instructors were trying to cause the students to be single-minded on where they stood. When I spoke with the one instructor to try to change the program to fit me so that I could succeed, I could not move forward from the place that I was, until I chose to continue. I'm going to rephrase this. When I tried to control the situation because it caused me to *fear failing*, it was not until I took a single-minded position on where I stood and resolved in my mind to continue, that I actually moved forward. In James 1:8, we see that: "A double minded man is unstable in all his ways." My trying to control the situation, in of an act of desperation, revealed the fear that was in my heart. Fear is exact opposite of faith. 2 Timothy 1:7 tells us that: "God has not given us a spirit of fear; but of love, power, and of a sound mind." Matthew 8:24-26 shows us how the disciples responded to the tempest of the sea. They ran to Jesus believing that they were perishing. The Scripture tells us in verse 26 how Jesus responded to them: "And he said to them, why are ye fearful, o ye of little faith? Then He arose and rebuked the winds and the sea; and there was a great calm."

I shared with you that an instructor in the Psych Program encouraged us to put our thoughts in order daily. It was not until later, after the program adventure that the Holy Spirit showed me what she was actually saying. The clinical rotation in which she said this to us was a state hospital. I don't think that she was free to teach the word of God there openly; however, she was telling us to judge our thoughts. Philippians 4:8 shows us: "Whatsoever things are true, whatsoever things are honest, whatsoever things are just, whatsoever things are pure, whatsoever things are lovely, whatsoever things are of good report, if there be any virtue, and if there be any praise, to think on these things." If the thoughts of the day were not true, honest, just, pure, lovely, and so on, we should deal with them.

She was encouraging us to "CAST DOWN IMAGINATIONS, and every high thing that exalteth itself against the knowledge of God, and to BRING INTO CAPTIVITY every thought to the obedience of Christ," from 2 Corinthians 10:5. She did not actually say it, but I know in my spirit she was telling us to bring every thought into kingdom order. Keeping our hearts with all diligence for out of them are the issues of life and not letting our hearts be troubled.

Chapter 5

STAY IN YOUR LANE!

A TIMELY SLOGAN

You have probably heard "stay in your own lane" at one time or another. You may have even used the saying yourself. It's a metaphor of correction to people who are poking their noses into things that have nothing to do with them. The metaphor implies that a person can not drive two cars at the same time or one car in two lanes. It also implies that a person can not run a race in his own lane and someone else's at the same time without the possibility of disaster. The disaster could be as simple as someone not being where they need to be when they need to be there, or totally tripping up or jamming up the second lane that they are wrongfully trying to possess. Either way, it's about being a busybody. I know that it seems as though I have come out of a bag on you here; but I am calling it what it is. The question that I would ask here is, what are you supposed to be doing? More specifically, what is the Lord of Hosts instructing you to do? Do that.

Many times a believer may have a directive from the Lord, and, as they look at it, they may sense things that would not want them to follow through with that instruction. Doubt wants to be one such hindrance. If a person comes into agreement

21

with doubt, he could tell himself, "God could not mean for me to do this, or the Lord of Hosts could not want to move through me like that." Why not? He is no respecter of persons. Why not you? I remember years ago, when the Lord began to increase the gifts of His Spirit to me. I was driving, and the Lord told me something in another tongue by His Spirit. The Lord then began to give me the interpretation, and, as He did, doubt surrounded my mind to hinder my focus on what the Lord was telling me. Immediately the Lord said, "Don't take your eyes off of me to look at doubt!" This was a new thing for me, and Holy Spirit was instructing me. In 1 Corinthians 12: 8-10, we see the spiritual gifts. The gift of interpretation of tongues was new to me.

Fear of man wants to be another hindrance. If a person comes into agreement with this fear of man thing, he could ask himself, "What will people think if I do what God is telling me to do?" Fear of man wants to cause a person to possibly conjure up scenarios for the outcome of their obedience to what God has told them to do.

Unbelief wants to be another hindrance. A person may believe in God the Father and Yeshua the King of kings, but not believe in what He will do. Maybe it's unbelief in what He can do. Whichever it is, I can't want it because it wants to hinder what the Sovereign Ruler of the universe does through me. I can't want that. I won't come into agreement with it.

We have already established that the mind is the main arena of battle. In 2 Corinthians 10:5, we have an instruction: "Casting down IMAGINATIONS, and every high thing that exalteth itself against the knowledge of God, and bringing into captivity every thought to the obedience of Christ." I don't believe that I can say this one too much, it is just that important to let the mind of Christ be in us. We also see in Psalms 19:14 David asking the Lord, "Let the words of my mouth and the meditation of my heart be acceptable in thy sight, O Lord, my strength, and my redeemer."

Let's look at this...*the words of my mouth*. In Proverbs 18:21, we see that: "Death and life are in the power of the tongue: and they that love it shall eat the fruit thereof." Let's break it down more. The meditation of my heart, Proverbs 4:23, shows us that the issues of life flow from our hearts and that we are to keep it diligently. You may ask, "How do we keep our hearts?" If it is not good, pure, or holy don't meditate on it. You may say, "But my mind and my heart are separate." Proverbs 23:7 instructs us that, "For as he THINKETH in his heart, so is he." King Jesus asked the scribes, "why think ye evil in your hearts?" We see this in Matthew 9:4.

You see the King of kings is very concerned with our hearts. I want to be very transparent with you here. Fear of man would want to stop me from writing some of the things that I am writing right now. I say to that, "Let God be true but every man a liar." Romans3:4. I stand in boldness to write what has been placed in my spirit to tell you. In Romans 3:3, Paul asks, "For what if some did not believe? Shall their unbelief make the faith of God without effect?"

Writing this book is obedience unto God the Father. He spoke of it back in 1999-2000, and until now I have been walking the book out. I am now putting it on paper. When the Lord confirmed that it was time for this book to come forth, I asked Him, "Really Lord, another self-help book?" I have since grasped the mindset that if only one person is helped through this book, then so be it. I just want to stay in my lane and do what the Lord is telling me to do when He tells me to do it, even if that one person is me. I may sound conceited, but please don't get confidence twisted with conceit. I have faith that the Lord knows my lying down and my uprising. I believe that He knows me altogether, has fashioned me, and directs my path. Did you note that I said *I believe*? I have faith that these things are so.

In the book of John 15:13-15, Jesus is telling His disciples how He loved them with the greatest of love by giving His life for his friends. He then says that we are His friends if we keep His command. I say, "Yes," to whatever the command may be. He then says that we are friends because whatever He hears of the Father He makes known to us. That truth about my Savior is lovingly precious to me.

What do you do if you want to become friends with someone? I personally may talk to that person and listen to them. I can learn things about this person if I listen to them. I may try spending time with them. At this point, I am showing them that I really want to get to know them. Once I begin to know what offends them, I probably don't want to do that because this friendship is valuable to me. If I gain knowledge into what they like, I will probably do those things because, once again, this friendship is valuable to me.

It is like this with our Lord and Savior. The only thing that is different is, it must be done in spirit and in truth. He is all-knowing; so you can't come half-steppin'. You have got to come with your heart wide open. In Psalms 139:3-6, David is speaking on how the Lord God is acquainted with all of his ways. He speaks of how the Lord knows every word on his tongue and how His hand is upon him. He then says a key thing: "Such knowledge is too wonderful for me; it is high, I cannot attain unto it." God's knowledge, God's ways, His heart, even God's will cannot be attained on our own. I agree with the psalmist David—His thoughts are beyond us. We have available to us the Spirit of truth who teaches us all things, leads us into all truths, and searches the deep things of God, we may know the heart of God. It is by His Spirit.

Like never before, people are seeking to move in the spirit realm. God the Father has placed a hunger in men to move out of their fleshly actions and move in Him by His Spirit. We must remember that those who are led by the Spirit of God are the sons of God. The thing that I have seen is people trying to mix the things of God with the things of Satan.

Marvin Sapp in his song, "You are God alone," says it perfectly, "If you are looking for somebody, He's God; and He don't need nobody else." I will take it further and say, "He don't need nothing else." We don't need God the Father and Wicca. We don't need God the Father and white magic, or God the Father and third eye open. We just need to come out of our comfort zones to where the Great I Am is calling us. He is all that we need Him to be. We have to get to know Him deeply. In the last part of Daniel 11:32, it is written, "But the people that know their God shall be strong and do exploits." We have got to get to know Him for ourselves.

Now let me get back to the lanes. We have a great cloud of witnesses. The book of Hebrews tells us that it is the saints that have gone on to be with the Lord. Glory! My mother always told us that we could do anything. She even prayed that everything that our hands touched would prosper. To know, that now, she finally sees me running this race that has been set before me is encouraging.

When a runner is trying to do his best, he usually does not want to be weighed down. He even wears clothing that is lightweight. Hebrews 12:1 shows us how, "Wherefore seeing that we also are compassed with so great a cloud of witnesses, let us lay aside every weight and sin which doth so easily beset us, and let us run with patience the race that has been set before us." Hmmm.

We talked earlier about things that want to try to hinder our obedience to the King of kings. You see, He came and walked this walk before us and made the path clear. We have but to walk it all the way. Some weights that want to slow a believer down may be the things that I spoke of earlier—like fear, unbelief, or pride; there could be so many things that want to hinder obedience. If a person is in agreement with fear, when God says for them to move, they may not. If a person has come into agreement with pride, and God says, "No, not that way," that person may lean on his own understanding, do it their way and fall. This walk will not appeal to our intellect or comfort; however, Jesus the King of kings has already done it and the Holy Spirit knows how to lead us through. In Matthew 11:29-30, Jesus tells us, "Take my yoke upon you and learn of me: for I am meek and lowly in heart: and ye shall find rest unto your soul, for my yoke is easy and my burden light."

I remember a dream that I had one morning. I was at this military command post of some sort. I was there with two other people, and we were looking for some type of official. We asked this woman about Him and she said a few things to us then went to get Him. Many things took place in this dream, but one thing I remember clearly is that, as we waited for this official to come, I saw to my right that there was this man with an out-of-this-world physique. He was seated, so I only saw him from the waist up. You have to understand that, being a bodybuilder, I have seen numerous of grand physiques; however, this one was out-of-this-world awesome. He had on a t-shirt with a black, grey, and white camouflage design that had silver literally traveling through it. When I looked at this guy's t-shirt, my eyes must have bucked or looked with a child-like *WOW!* His shirt moved as if it were alive. I could tell that he was chiseled with a tiny waist, even through the t-shirt. As I looked in amazement, he flashed the most joyous smile from ear to ear. Right after that, I was flung outside into a race. It was the kind of race set up that marathon runners are in: everyone all bunched up together. These people had a sense of humor because, when it was time to run, they told everyone around me to close me in. When I saw that they were playing a joke on me, I fell to the ground laughing. It was a very joyous atmosphere. I believe that the one in the camo with the joyous smile was an angel of the Lord's. I believe that I was there to get direction from the Commander in Chief (Jesus). I did not see Him; however there is just this *knowing* in my spirit. I also believe that it was Jesus that slung me back into the race with a new attitude. In that time, I was standing and believing God for some things. I did not know it, but my eyes had begun to focus on circumstances around what I believed God for. Focus has to remain on Yeshua the King of kings; if not, one may begin to sink when Jesus says, *come walk with Me on the ocean.* Although there were no lanes in that night vision, there was a direction. The Lord had been talking to me about my attitude. He adjusted it and showed me the power of walking in His joy.

I said before that Jesus has asked us to learn of Him; His burden is light. We have to stay focused on Him and not on the one in the next lane. We can't focus on the next man's shoes, the next man's pace, the next man's gifts or anointing. We have to focus on Jesus. The Holy Spirit will pace us to be in sync with His will and the timing for things that He has planned. This also takes obedience for us to walk circumspectly and not get in a hurry or drag our feet. That obedience is immediate and exact.

In the book of John, Jesus speaks to Peter and prophesies to him; then, Jesus tells Peter "Follow me." John 21:19. Now Peter looks at John and is wondering as well as asking Jesus, "Lord, what will this man do?" Jesus said, "If I will that he tarry til I come, what is that to thee? Follow thou me." John 21:21, 22. Basically even Jesus is telling us to stay in our own lane.

Chapter 6

THE CALL TO COACH LIFE!

I must tell you that it has truly been a joy to write these testimonies and share about the life that God the Father has
given me. It has been a joy to share some of the ways that He
has expressed Himself to me over the years. It is truly a wonder.
I am positive that greater expressions and manifestations of
Him are yet to come to me and through me. I shared with you
in an earlier chapter my response to the Father's instruction
to write this book. I didn't understand why, what I had to say
couldn't just be said in an individual testimony, but He did.
He knows exactly who needs what, and when. He also knows
how. I believe and rest in that truth with all of my being. In the
authority of son-ship of the Most High God, the authority that
Jesus made available for me, I stepped out and He met me. He
caused rivers of living water to flow from my belly to whoever
needed to hear what has been said here. Glory!

In 2003, I returned to Texas from California and had been
working in a personal training facility. The Lord began to
impress on me to move to another gym. This place that God
was moving me to, was a privately-owned powerhouse gym
where I trained myself when I was not training others at the
facility. I had spoken to the owner of this powerhouse back in
2001 about training people there, in his gym; however, he was

not open to the idea, and thus I worked at the other facility. When God the Father began to speak to my heart about moving, I was a little resistant. What would I do for clients? I had bills to pay and an eleven year old son to raise. Although the way was not yet clear to me, the Lord continued to prepare my heart on the matter.

One day I was at the powerhouse gym when the owner, (The same man that I had spoken to about personal training years before), walked up to me and began talking about a few people who wanted personal training there in his gym. He went on to say, "Of course you would have to be here," meaning *his* gym. Amazing, the same man who totally did not want to be bothered with it—the same man that just could not see how a person could make money training people—was there asking me to do that very thing in his gym. I considered but did not move until things just seemed to begin to close for me at my work place and point me to the door that the Lord was leading me to walk through. There were a few clients that God sent with me to the new location.

Now, I'm in a new gym with new hours, and what do I do? I go on vacation. It was the perfect time for me to go refocus and prepare for the newness. So many times we think that we know what's going on, and then sometimes God will allow us to see what's really going on. This trip was a time of relaxation; however, it was also a time of instruction. While on vacation the Lord told me, "You are no longer a personal trainer. You are a life coach." I said, "Um, okay. How do I do that?" He reminded me that He came that we have life and that we have it more abundantly. That's all that I really remember His saying about the call then.

Over the years to come, when someone would ask me, "What do you do?" I would answer them, "I'm a life coach." They would quickly come back with, "Oh you are a lifeguard? Okay." I would say, "No, I'm a life *coach*." They would look at me with a perplexed look on their face. As time went on, we began to see various types of life coaches emerge. We saw relational coaches, financial coaches, time management coaches, just to name a few. At that time when asked what I did and I answered life coached; the question was, "Oh, what kind of life coach are you?" These two scenarios of request for explanation of God's call caused me, in times past, to take the road most traveled. For years, I compromised my stance on what God the Father had spoken to me, by openly decreeing over myself that I was a personal trainer and life coach or a life coach and personal trainer. It would just depend on what I felt the person that I was speaking to at the time could understand. When the Lord called me to coach life, He said, "You are no longer a personal trainer, you are a life coach."

I remember when I first began to coach people under this new calling. I had a client who was going on a ski trip and had not planned on skiing, but would read most of the time while her family skied. I had a book on intercession that I had finished reading. The book was really meaty. I suggested it to her; and, on the day that I brought it to her, I said, "It's very meaty." She said, "Okay." I held on to the other end of the book as I continued to explain, "It's pretty intense." She looked at me and said, "Okay, you say that to me as if I can't handle intense. I train with you, I think I can handle intense." I said, "Yes but this is..." the Holy Spirit stopped me with an intense truth and redirection, He said, "You have permission to speak freely!" I let the book go, and that was the end of that moment.

I would like to take time to coach you for a moment. Is that okay? When the Lord tells us something, instructs us, calls us to something, He is always going to see it through—always. We have to guard our hearts and seek that the words of our mouth, our meditations, are pleasing to God. We want our thoughts to be in line with His heart and His will in everything. When the Lord told me that I had permission to speak freely, I had come into a new place spiritually, as well as physically. I was accustomed to working in places where one just avoids politics or a personal relationship with God as topics of discussion. The Father was setting up His marketplace ministry through me, and my thinking was getting in the way. He spoke the truth that I had permission to speak freely. His truth gave me a whole new perception on the thing. I began to live and move in Him in ways that I had never imagined I would in the workplace. All in all, it was Him through me. I know that we will pray to ourselves at our jobs or with co-workers. Maybe we pray when no one is around or even at home about work situations. The Lord has not only called me to be a secret agent, but also a bold ambassador for His Kingdom in the marketplace. He has called me to coach the whole man.

I once had a client that I was helping to attain a goal. One day during our training relationship, I was sharing a testimony with her. I got to a part where I shared that God the Father had spoken to me, and I told her that He had said *thus and thus*. This lady kind of paused and said, "He did..." She did not say it as a question but more like an unbelieving, "Hmm...sure He did." I saw that she was having trouble with even the thought of Abba Father talking to us. People sometimes have difficulty believing that He is even interested in communing with us. I said to her, "Yes, He did."

A few weeks later, I was training this same lady right in the middle of the gym. She had gotten into a mindset that, if she missed one day of cardio, all was lost. I told her that this was a lifestyle adaptation, and she would do this for the rest of her life. I encouraged her to not feel driven or defeated if one day she had to travel earlier than when she did cardio. She said she knew, but she just could not shake loose of it. I stepped up to her and simply said, "Then, as your life coach, I loose you from that mindset in the name of Jesus and decree liberty and freedom of life to you in this endeavor in Jesus name." She returned to her next set; and, as we stood there in the middle of that gym, a powerful, tangible presence of the Spirit of God flowed over us. The manifestation of His presence was so strong there that my client said, "I hope that this is Him." I said, "Yes, this is Him!" We just stayed there as God did what He wanted to do in us.

There was another instance in those days where God the Father flowed through me to speak truth that caused eyes to see from a liberated perception. A client was warming up on the elliptical. I walked up to greet her; I could sense a roaring (undercurrent) in her being. After warm up, I wanted to stretch her to prepare for the work to come, but she was in a mindset of "Come on, let's get to it." She asked me what we were going to do first, and I felt led to say, "Breathe. We are going to just breathe for a moment." This was a little uncomfortable for her, and she began to weep. It is not that the breathing was uncomfortable; it was the stopping and *being*. She began to share; and the Spirit of God met us there in the marketplace and brought peace, He brought truth. There are so many testimonies.

I have definitely dropped personal trainer from the description of what God does through me, and now I simply state that I am a life coach. It does not matter what any one thinks or says about it. What did God say? That's what matters.

I feel a need to remind you what life is. Jesus is life. In John 14:6, Jesus speaks to the disciples and says, "I am the way the truth, and the life: no man cometh unto the Father, but by me." I shared with you that, when the Lord called me to coach life and I asked Him how, He reminded me that He came that we have life and that we have it more abundantly.

Now this is what I see where I stand, He is life. Without Him, there is no life. Without Christ, there is just mere existence. I say this without hesitation because I have been there and have seen that. I know what it is and how it looks. He called me to coach life, and of the increase of His government and His peace there shall be no end. He has called me to decree His Kingdom come and His will be done, in whatever I see that is short of life. I'm not speaking of life as we think we know it, but life as He came that we might receive. It is the zeal of the Lord of Hosts that will perform this, not me. Abundant life is so vast that I truly can't touch the depth of it on my own; however, I am on a journey for more of God.

When Jesus was praying to the Father in John 17, in verse 3, Jesus said, "And this is life eternal, that they might know thee the only true God, and Jesus Christ, whom thou hast sent." He wants us to know Him intimately. You know the saying that you are known by the company that you keep? That is exactly what He wants. Jesus wants us to be known by keeping company with Him. I'm not saying that He does not want us to have other friends; however, I am saying that, as we keep company with Him, we will begin to know Him more. We will begin to see things from His perspective because we are being conformed to His image by Holy Spirit.

Please, right now if you have not received Jesus personally as your Lord and Savior, and you sense the Holy Spirit drawing you to Jesus with this strong desire to know Him, to be saved by Him, do so right now. Just tell Jesus that you realize that, as humans, we all have sinned, and that you repent for all of your sins and ask Him to forgive you. Tell Jesus that you believe that He came to give you life and you receive the life that He came to give you. Ask Jesus to come into your heart and be the Lord and Savior of your life forever. We all worship something; let it be the only true and living God. Maybe you have received Jesus as your Lord and Savior, but you just have not taken time to get to know Him. Is it possible that you couldn't see how this awesome God could be interested in spending time with you? He is, and He is so loving, actually He is Love. Right now, please, if this is you, just tell Him that you don't know how to "be" in Him, what does it mean to worship Him in Spirit and in truth? Ask Him. Tell the Holy Spirit, "I need you to teach me." Maybe you have received Jesus as your Savior but have never received the baptism of the Holy Ghost, the Spirit of truth who will lead you into all truths, teach you all things, and show you things to come. Let it be now just ask Him, "Holy Spirit, I need you to walk this walk in the abundant life that Jesus came to give me. I ask you to flow, flow, and flow into me Holy Spirit until I'm am filled with you to overflowing in Jesus' name."

I thank you Father for making provisions for me to become the righteousness of Christ.......Here I am on what seems a brink and a totter. All and all I know it is You on which I stand. If there should be a totter, it would be that I dipped my foot to sifting sand. We are here, Father, on oceans deep, grasping to post up on something that would feel like land...our faith, ministries? Those, too, are but sifting sand if not yielded to the Cornerstone of this body; His body, in Him, on Him is where we have been called to stand! So here I am Jesus, with all my desires...the ones given to me by You and the ones that linger in my heart! Here I am with all my gifts and gains. I lay them as humbly as I know how to, at your feet. I look into your eyes; I search for your heart! Please take my hand and lead me through the eye of this needle. If I must go it alone...then boldly, I stand to leap through it. For I can't make it with just *some* revelation of You. I must have all that You have for me. True to myself? That won't suffice! I must be true to You.